Ashley Fitzgerald

SOMATIC THERAPY FOR HYPERTENSION

Healing the Body and Calming the Mind to Lower Blood Pressure

Published by UNITEXTO

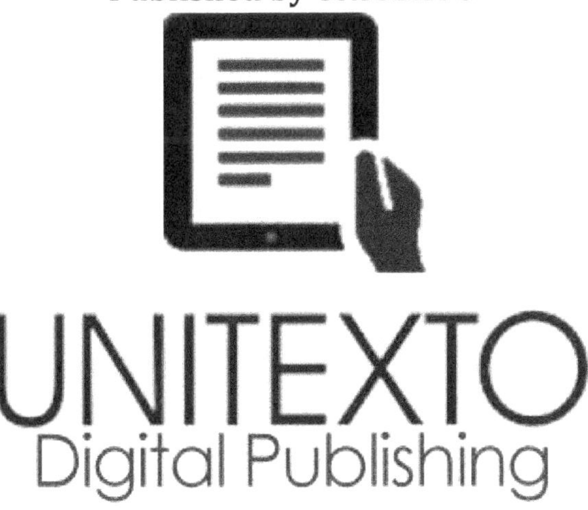

TABLE OF CONTENTS

- Mindfulness and its impact on hypertension.
- Body scanning and somatic experiencing.
- Developing a daily mindfulness practice.

Chapter 7: Emotional Regulation and Stress Management

- Understanding the impact of emotions on blood pressure.
- Techniques for managing stress and emotional responses.
- The role of therapy and counseling.

Chapter 8: Diet, Lifestyle, and Hypertension

- The role of diet in managing hypertension.
- Importance of physical activity.
- Lifestyle modifications to support somatic practices.

Chapter 9: Integrating Somatic Therapy into Daily Life

- Developing a daily somatic routine.
- Overcoming challenges and staying motivated.
- Case studies and success stories.

Chapter 10: Future Directions and Research

- Emerging research in somatic therapy for hypertension.
- Integrating somatic practices with medical treatment.
- The future of holistic approaches to hypertension management.

Chapter 11. Daily routine recommended

Chapter 12. Reference

-Books
-Academic research

Why this book?

In today's fast-paced world, the prevalence of hypertension continues to rise, posing a significant health risk to millions worldwide. As the silent killer lurking beneath the surface, hypertension demands our attention and a multifaceted approach to management.

"Somatic Therapy for Hypertension: Healing the Body and Calming the Mind to Lower Blood Pressure" delves into the depths of somatic practices, offering a beacon of hope for those seeking holistic solutions to this pervasive health challenge. This book emerges from the pressing need to explore alternative avenues for hypertension management, ones that transcend conventional medical treatments to embrace the interconnectedness of the mind and body.

By bridging the gap between somatic therapy and cardiovascular health, this book aims to empower readers with practical tools, evidence-based strategies, and a newfound sense of agency over their well-being. Join us on a journey of self-discovery and transformation as we navigate the realms of somatic healing and cardiovascular wellness.

This is why you should buy and read this book:

1. **Holistic Approach:**
    "Somatic Therapy for Hypertension" takes a holistic approach to managing hypertension by addressing both the physical and psychological aspects of the condition. Readers will gain valuable insights into how somatic practices can complement traditional medical treatments,

leading to a more comprehensive approach to hypertension management.

2. **Evidence-Based Strategies:**
Backed by research and clinical evidence, this book provides readers with evidence-based somatic therapy techniques that have been proven to lower blood pressure and improve cardiovascular health. Each strategy is explained in detail, allowing readers to understand the underlying mechanisms and benefits.

3. **Practical Guidance:**
With practical exercises, mindfulness techniques, and breathing practices, this book offers readers actionable tools to incorporate somatic therapy into their daily lives. Whether you're new to somatic practices or experienced in mind-body approaches, the book provides clear guidance suitable for all levels.

4. **Empowerment and Self-Care:**
By learning somatic therapy techniques, readers can take an active role in managing their hypertension and promoting their overall well-being. The book empowers readers to become active participants in their health journey, fostering a sense of self-efficacy and autonomy.

5. **Improved Quality of Life:**
Beyond symptom management, "Somatic Therapy for Hypertension" emphasizes the importance of holistic wellness and the interconnectedness of mind, body, and spirit. By incorporating somatic practices into their daily

routine, readers can not only lower their blood pressure but also enhance their overall health, resilience, and quality of life.

Take control of your hypertension journey and embark on a path to holistic wellness with "Somatic Therapy for Hypertension." Empower yourself with evidence-based somatic practices proven to lower blood pressure, reduce stress, and promote cardiovascular health.

Say goodbye to the limitations of traditional treatments and embrace a comprehensive approach that nurtures both your body and mind. Start your journey toward optimal health today and discover the transformative power of somatic healing.

Ashley Fitzgerald

About the Author:

Ashley Fitzgerald: An Embodiment of Healing and Personal Triumph
From a tender age, I, Ashley Fitzgerald, was acutely attuned to the nuances of health and personal well-being. These early inklings of self-awareness were not just passing contemplations but the seeds of a lifelong journey towards self-improvement and healing.

As the chapters of life unfolded, I embraced my calling with fervor, transforming my youthful concerns into a robust career that spans two decades. Today, I stand before you not merely as a practitioner but as a seasoned professional healer whose hands and heart have been instrumental in guiding countless individuals towards weight loss triumphs, enriched sexual health, and the surmounting of life's multifaceted challenges to reach the pinnacle of their health aspirations.

My professional and academic journey is a tapestry of diverse yet interconnected disciplines. With an insatiable thirst for knowledge, I delved deep into the realms of yoga and meditation, not just as practices but as academic pursuits, seeking to understand their profound effects on the human psyche and physiology.

This spiritual and intellectual quest further led me to the healing energies of Reiki, the organic wisdom in health foods, and the transformative potential of neuroscience and positive psychology.

My foray into the science of health and exercise is not merely academic; it is a reflection of my intrinsic philosophy that the body and mind are inextricable partners in the dance of life.

My dedication to personal growth extends beyond my professional endeavors—it is a way of life. Each morning, as the world stirs awake, I find sanctuary in my daily rituals. My practice of yoga is more than a physical regimen; it is a journey towards achieving a state of zen-like tranquility, a testament to my belief in the power of simplicity and inner peace. Meditation accompanies yoga as my mental compass, guiding me through life's tumultuous waves with a steadfast calm.

What fuels my unyielding passion is an unwavering drive—an innate desire to not only absorb the myriad teachings that life has to offer but also to disseminate them. I am imbued with a relentless drive to unearth and share life strategies that spark a transformative flame within souls, urging them to reach for health, well-being, and the fruition of their deepest dreams.

It was this very desire that led me to the world of writing, to become a scribe of my experiences and insights. My pen is driven by a profound commitment to be a beacon of positivity, influencing the lives of others through words that resonate with truth and vitality.

As you turn the pages of my books, what you will find is a reflection of my heart's work. I invite you into my world, not just as a reader, but as a fellow traveler on this grand adventure of life. Thank you for embarking on this journey with me, and it is my sincerest hope that you will find as much joy in reading my writings as I found in penning them down. May the words you peruse inspire you to cultivate the health and happiness you so richly deserve.

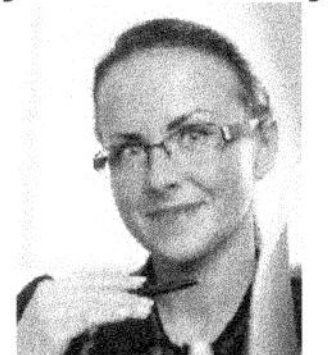

Ashley Fitzgerald

Chapter 1: Understanding Hypertension

- Definition and overview of hypertension.
- Causes and risk factors.
- Effects of hypertension on health and wellbeing.

Definition and Overview of Hypertension

Hypertension, commonly known as high blood pressure, is a medical condition where the force of the blood against the artery walls is consistently too high. Blood pressure is determined by both the amount of blood the heart pumps and the resistance to blood flow in the arteries. It's typically defined by blood pressure readings above 140/90 mmHg, and more recently, 130/80 mmHg according to the American Heart Association. Understanding hypertension is crucial, as it is often a silent condition, going unnoticed until it causes significant health issues.

Hypertension is categorized into two types: primary (essential) hypertension and secondary hypertension. Primary hypertension develops over time with no identifiable cause and is the most common type. Secondary hypertension, on the other hand, results from an underlying condition, such as kidney disease or endocrine disorders, and tends to appear suddenly.

Causes and Risk Factors

The exact causes of primary hypertension are not entirely understood, but several factors and conditions may play a role:

1. Genetics:

A family history of hypertension increases the likelihood of developing it.

2. Age:
    The risk increases as you age, particularly after age 65.
3. Race:
    Hypertension is more common in African American adults than in Caucasian or Hispanic American adults.
4. Lifestyle Choices:
    Poor diet (especially high in sodium), lack of physical activity, and consumption of alcohol and tobacco.
5. Obesity:
    Excess body weight can lead to hypertension by increasing the strain on the heart and arteries.
6. Stress:
    Chronic stress can contribute to hypertension, as can stress-related behaviors like eating unhealthy foods or drinking alcohol.

Secondary hypertension can be caused by conditions that affect the kidneys, arteries, heart, or endocrine system. Medications, including birth control pills, cold remedies, decongestants, pain relievers, and some prescription drugs, can also cause secondary hypertension.

Effects of Hypertension on Health and Wellbeing

Hypertension can lead to a range of health problems, some of which can be life-threatening. The increased pressure can cause damage to the arteries, heart, brain, kidneys, and eyes.

1. Heart and Artery Damage:
   Hypertension can lead to hardening and thickening of the arteries (atherosclerosis), which can result in a heart attack, stroke, or other complications.
2. Heart Failure:
   The increased workload from high blood pressure can cause the heart to enlarge and fail to supply blood to the body.
3. Brain Health:
   It can cause strokes, transient ischemic attacks (TIAs), and possibly dementia due to reduced blood flow to the brain.
4. Kidney Disease:
   The kidneys filter excess fluid and waste from the blood—a process that depends on healthy blood vessels. High blood pressure can injure both the blood vessels in and leading to the kidneys, causing several types of kidney disease (nephropathy).
5. Eye Health:
   Hypertension can cause damage to the blood vessels in the retina, potentially leading to blindness.

Apart from these physical health issues, hypertension can also significantly impact a person's mental health and overall wellbeing. The stress of managing a chronic condition can lead to anxiety, depression, and a diminished quality of life. Moreover, the medication's side effects and the dietary and lifestyle changes necessary to manage the condition can also affect a person's mental health.

In conclusion, hypertension is a complex condition with various causes and significant health impacts. Understanding its nature, causes, and effects is the first step in managing and treating it effectively. The following chapters will delve deeper into how somatic therapy can be an integral part of managing this condition, offering a holistic approach to health and wellness.

Chapter 2: Introduction to Somatic Therapy

- Definition and principles of somatic therapy.
- How somatic therapy differs from traditional therapies.
- Overview of somatic practices.
 Definition and Principles of Somatic Therapy

Definition and principles of somatic therapy

Somatic Therapy is a holistic therapeutic approach that emphasizes the connection between the mind and body in healing. The word "somatic" is derived from the Greek word "soma," which means the living body. This therapy recognizes that trauma and stress can manifest physically in the body's tissues and muscles. The primary principle of somatic therapy is the integration and synchronization of mind, body, spirit, and emotion for complete healing.

The core principles of somatic therapy include:

1. Body Awareness:
   It focuses on increasing the individual's awareness of their body, recognizing the sensations and experiences that reside within.
2. Mind-Body Connection:
   Acknowledging how the mind influences the body and vice versa, particularly how emotional and psychological factors can impact physical health.
3. Holistic Healing:
   Aims to treat the individual as a whole rather than just addressing specific symptoms or illnesses.
4. Empowerment and Autonomy:

Encouraging clients to discover their ability to self-regulate and heal, thereby gaining greater control over their health and wellbeing.

How Somatic Therapy Differs from Traditional Therapies

Somatic therapy differs from traditional therapies in several key ways:

1. Embodied Healing: Unlike traditional talk therapy, which primarily engages the cognitive aspects of healing, somatic therapy involves the physical body in the therapeutic process. It believes that the body holds onto past traumas and stress, which are expressed through physical symptoms.
2. Experiential Approach: Somatic therapy is more experiential, involving movement, touch, breathwork, and other physical exercises to release stored tension and trauma.
3. Client-Centered Therapy: It is highly individualized, focusing on the client's unique experiences and body responses, rather than following a standardized protocol.
4. Integration of Physical and Mental Health: Somatic therapy bridges the gap between mental and physical health, addressing both psychological and physiological aspects concurrently.

Overview of Somatic Practices

Somatic therapy encompasses a range of practices, each focusing on reconnecting the individual with their bodily sensations and experiences:

1. Body Awareness Techniques:
   Techniques such as mindfulness and body scanning help clients become more aware of bodily sensations and the emotions associated with them.
2. Breathing Exercises:
   Used to regulate the autonomic nervous system, reduce stress, and improve emotional regulation.
3. Movement Therapies: Practices like yoga, Tai Chi, or dance therapy, which use gentle movements to release tension and improve body awareness.
4. Biodynamic Craniosacral Therapy:
   A gentle practice focusing on the rhythms and movements of the craniosacral system to enhance body regulation and healing.
5. Myofascial Release:
   A hands-on technique that involves applying gentle sustained pressure into the myofascial connective tissue to eliminate pain and restore motion.

Each of these practices aids in releasing the physical manifestations of stress and trauma, fostering a holistic sense of well-being. The subsequent chapters will explore how these somatic practices can be specifically applied to managing hypertension, offering a comprehensive approach that complements traditional medical treatments.

Chapter 3: The Mind-Body Connection in Hypertension

- Exploring how mental and emotional states affect blood pressure.
- Stress and its impact on hypertension.
- The role of the autonomic nervous system.

Exploring How Mental and Emotional States Affect Blood Pressure

The mind and body are intricately connected, and this connection plays a crucial role in the regulation of blood pressure. Mental and emotional states can significantly influence blood pressure levels, either directly or indirectly. For instance, emotions such as anxiety, anger, or sadness can lead to temporary spikes in blood pressure. Over time, these repeated spikes may contribute to sustained high blood pressure.

The impact of mental health on hypertension is also evident. Conditions like depression and anxiety are often linked with higher rates of hypertension. This relationship is bidirectional; not only can mental health issues lead to increased blood pressure, but living with hypertension can also cause or exacerbate mental health problems due to the stress and anxiety related to managing a chronic condition.

Stress and Its Impact on Hypertension

Stress is a significant factor in the development and exacerbation of hypertension. When stressed, the body produces a surge of hormones which temporarily increase blood pressure by causing the heart to beat faster and the blood vessels to narrow. There are two types of stress: acute stress, which is short-lived, and chronic stress, which is prolonged and can be particularly harmful.

Chronic stress can lead to a consistently elevated blood pressure level. Moreover, the behaviors people adopt in response to stress, such as smoking, unhealthy eating, and excessive alcohol consumption, can further contribute to the development of hypertension.

The Role of the Autonomic Nervous System

The autonomic nervous system (ANS) plays a vital role in the regulation of blood pressure. It consists of two main components: the sympathetic nervous system (SNS) and the parasympathetic nervous system (PNS). The SNS is often referred to as the "fight or flight" system, which prepares the body for action, including increasing the heart rate and blood pressure. Conversely, the PNS is responsible for the "rest and digest" functions, slowing the heart rate and lowering blood pressure.

In individuals with hypertension, the balance between these two systems can be disrupted, often with an overactive SNS and an underactive PNS. This imbalance can lead to sustained high blood pressure. Stress, anxiety, and emotional turmoil can exacerbate this imbalance, further affecting blood pressure levels.

Therefore, managing mental and emotional health is crucial in the treatment and management of hypertension. Techniques that promote relaxation and stress reduction, such as those found in somatic therapy, can help in regulating the autonomic nervous system, thereby potentially reducing blood pressure levels. The following chapters will delve deeper into specific somatic practices and how they can be utilized to manage hypertension effectively, highlighting the critical role of the mind-body connection in overall health.

Chapter 4: Somatic Techniques for Relaxation

- Breathing exercises and their benefits.
- Progressive muscle relaxation.
- Guided imagery and visualization
 Breathing Exercises and Their Benefits

Breathing exercises and their benefits

Breathing exercises are a fundamental aspect of somatic therapy, particularly in managing hypertension. These exercises involve consciously controlling the breath to induce relaxation. Deep, slow breathing is known to activate the parasympathetic nervous system (PNS), which helps lower heart rate and blood pressure. Techniques such as diaphragmatic breathing, where breaths are deep and the belly expands, can be especially effective.

Benefits of breathing exercises include:

- Reduction of Stress:
They help in reducing stress and anxiety, which are significant contributors to hypertension.
- Regulation of Blood Pressure:
By activating the PNS, these exercises can help in naturally lowering blood pressure.
- Improved Oxygenation:
 Deep breathing enhances oxygen exchange, which is beneficial for overall cardiovascular health.
- Enhanced Body Awareness:
Practicing controlled breathing increases awareness of the body's responses and needs.

Progressive Muscle Relaxation

Progressive muscle relaxation (PMR) is another effective somatic technique. It involves tensing and then relaxing different muscle groups in the body. This practice helps in identifying and releasing tension held in the muscles. PMR can be particularly beneficial for individuals with hypertension, as it aids in reducing overall stress and tension levels.

The benefits of PMR include:

- Reduced Muscle Tension:
Helps in lowering the physical effects of stress, including muscle tension that can contribute to high blood pressure.
- Mind-Body Connection:
Enhances the connection between physical sensations and mental states, promoting holistic well-being.
- Stress and Anxiety Reduction:
By focusing on relaxing the muscles, the mind also relaxes, reducing feelings of stress and anxiety.
- Improved Sleep Quality:
PMR can lead to better sleep, which is crucial for maintaining healthy blood pressure levels.

Guided Imagery and Visualization

Guided imagery and visualization are techniques that involve focusing the mind on positive, calming images and scenarios. This practice can significantly impact the body's stress response, reducing the production of stress hormones that elevate blood pressure.

The benefits of guided imagery include:

- Enhanced Relaxation:
By mentally transporting to a peaceful place, the body responds with a reduction in heart rate and blood pressure.
- Emotional Regulation:
 It can help in managing emotions, an essential factor in controlling hypertension.
- Cognitive Distraction:
 Offers a mental diversion from stressors, providing temporary relief from chronic stress.
- Improved Autonomic Regulation:
 Can help in rebalancing the autonomic nervous system, essential for managing hypertension.

Incorporating these somatic relaxation techniques into daily life can be a powerful tool in managing hypertension. They offer a non-pharmacological approach to reduce blood pressure and improve overall well-being. The subsequent chapters will further explore how these practices can be integrated into a comprehensive approach to hypertension management, focusing on practical applications and real-life examples.

Chapter 5: Movement-Based Somatic Practices
- Gentle yoga and stretching for hypertension.
- Tai Chi and Qigong.
- The role of posture and alignment. Gentle Yoga and Stretching for Hypertension

- Gentle yoga and stretching for hypertension

Gentle yoga and stretching exercises are excellent movement-based somatic practices that can help in managing hypertension. Yoga combines physical postures, breathing exercises, and meditation to enhance overall health. For those with hypertension, gentle yoga styles such as Hatha or Yin Yoga are particularly beneficial. These styles focus on slow movements, deep stretches, and relaxation.

Benefits of gentle yoga and stretching include:

- Reduced Blood Pressure:
Yoga can help lower blood pressure by promoting relaxation and reducing stress.
- Improved Flexibility and Strength:
These practices enhance physical fitness, which is beneficial for cardiovascular health.
- Enhanced Mind-Body Awareness:
Yoga encourages mindfulness, which can help in recognizing and managing stress triggers.
- Balanced Autonomic Nervous System:
 Yoga helps balance the sympathetic and parasympathetic nervous systems, crucial for blood pressure regulation.

Tai Chi and Qigong

Tai Chi and Qigong are ancient Chinese practices that combine slow, deliberate movements with deep breathing and mental focus. These practices are particularly suitable for people with hypertension as they are low-impact and focus on relaxation and smooth flow of movements.

The benefits of Tai Chi and Qigong include:

- Stress Reduction:
The meditative movement helps in reducing stress and anxiety, which are key factors in managing hypertension.
- Improved Cardiovascular Health:
Regular practice can improve heart health and circulation, potentially lowering blood pressure.
- Enhanced Balance and Stability:
These practices strengthen the muscles and improve balance, which is beneficial for overall physical health.
- Boosted Immune Function:
Tai Chi and Qigong are known to enhance overall health, including immune function.

The Role of Posture and Alignment

Proper posture and alignment are crucial in movement-based somatic practices. Poor posture can lead to muscle tension, pain, and imbalances in the body, which can indirectly affect blood pressure. On the other hand, good posture ensures proper alignment of bones and muscles, reduces strain on the body, and improves breathing and circulation.

Key aspects include:

- Reduced Muscle Strain and Tension:
 Proper posture reduces the strain on muscles and
joints, leading to overall physical comfort.
- Improved Breathing:
Good alignment enhances lung capacity and breathing
efficiency, which is vital for stress management and
blood pressure regulation.
- Enhanced Body Awareness:
Focusing on posture increases bodily awareness,
helping individuals recognize and correct imbalances.

Integrating these movement-based somatic practices
into a daily routine can offer significant benefits for
individuals with hypertension. They not only address
the physical aspects of high blood pressure but also the
mental and emotional factors. The next chapters will
delve deeper into how these practices can be applied
effectively for hypertension management, providing
guidelines and real-world applications.

Chapter 6: Body Awareness and Mindfulness

- Mindfulness and its impact on hypertension.
- Body scanning and somatic experiencing.
- Developing a daily mindfulness practice.
  Mindfulness and Its Impact on Hypertension

- Mindfulness and its impact on hypertension

Mindfulness, a practice of maintaining a nonjudgmental state of heightened or complete awareness of one's thoughts, emotions, or experiences on a moment-to-moment basis, can have a profound impact on hypertension. This practice helps in managing stress, a major contributing factor to high blood pressure. By fostering a calm, focused state of mind, mindfulness can reduce the activation of the sympathetic nervous system, which is responsible for the body's 'fight or flight' response that raises blood pressure.

Benefits of mindfulness in managing hypertension include:

- Stress Reduction:
Regular mindfulness practice helps in reducing stress, a significant trigger for hypertension.
- Improved Emotional Regulation:
It aids in managing emotions effectively, reducing the likelihood of stress-induced hypertension.
- Enhanced Autonomic Balance:
 Mindfulness can contribute to balancing the sympathetic and parasympathetic nervous systems, vital for blood pressure regulation.
- Increased Awareness:

It increases awareness of lifestyle habits that may contribute to high blood pressure, such as diet and physical activity.

Body Scanning and Somatic Experiencing

Body scanning is a mindfulness technique where attention is moved through various parts of the body to identify and release tension. Somatic experiencing, on the other hand, is a therapeutic approach that focuses on bodily sensations to heal trauma and stress. Both techniques can be particularly effective for individuals with hypertension as they encourage deep relaxation and stress release.

The benefits of these practices include:

- Release of Muscle Tension:
They help in identifying and releasing stored tension in the body, which can contribute to high blood pressure.
- Enhanced Body Awareness:
These practices improve body awareness, helping individuals recognize the physical signs of stress and tension.
- Emotional Release:
They can facilitate the release of pent-up emotions, potentially lowering stress-induced physiological responses.

Developing a Daily Mindfulness Practice

Incorporating mindfulness into daily life is crucial for long-term management of hypertension. This can involve setting aside time each day for mindfulness exercises, such as meditation, deep breathing, or body scanning. It can also mean practicing mindfulness in everyday activities, like eating, walking, or even during work.

Strategies for developing a daily mindfulness practice include:

- Routine Practice:
Setting a specific time each day for mindfulness activities.
- Mindful Activities:
Engaging in activities that naturally encourage mindfulness, such as gardening, painting, or cooking.
- Mindfulness Apps and Resources:
Utilizing digital resources like apps or online programs for guided mindfulness exercises.
- Mindful Moments:
Taking short breaks throughout the day to practice deep breathing or to simply observe one's thoughts and sensations.

Through consistent practice, mindfulness can significantly contribute to managing hypertension. Not only does it offer a non-pharmacological approach to lowering blood pressure, but it also enhances overall well-being and quality of life. The next chapters will explore further applications of somatic therapies in the context of hypertension, offering practical advice and guidance for integrating these practices into everyday life.

Chapter 7: Emotional Regulation and Stress Management

- Understanding the impact of emotions on blood pressure.
- Techniques for managing stress and emotional responses.
- The role of therapy and counseling.
 Understanding the Impact of Emotions on Blood Pressure

- Understanding the impact of emotions on blood pressure.

Emotions play a significant role in the regulation of blood pressure. Emotional responses, particularly those like anger, anxiety, and stress, can cause temporary spikes in blood pressure. Over time, if these emotional states are chronic or recurrent, they can contribute to long-term hypertension. The physiological response to strong emotions often involves the release of stress hormones, like adrenaline and cortisol, which temporarily increase heart rate and constrict blood vessels, leading to higher blood pressure.

Key points include:

- Immediate Impact:
Emotional arousal can lead to immediate, though temporary, increases in blood pressure.
- Chronic Effects:
Chronic emotional stress or instability can contribute to sustained high blood pressure.
- Mind-Body Connection:

The physiological responses to emotions highlight the interconnectedness of emotional health and physical health, particularly cardiovascular health.

Techniques for Managing Stress and Emotional Responses

Managing stress and emotional responses is crucial in controlling hypertension. Several techniques and practices can be employed to achieve this:

1. Deep Breathing and Relaxation Techniques: These help to calm the mind and reduce the physiological effects of stress.
2. Regular Physical Activity: Exercise is a powerful stress reducer. It helps in releasing endorphins, the body's natural mood lifters.
3. Mindfulness and Meditation: These practices aid in developing a more balanced emotional state, reducing the likelihood of stress-induced blood pressure spikes.
4. Cognitive Behavioral Therapy (CBT): This is a form of psychotherapy that helps in changing negative thought patterns that contribute to stress and emotional turmoil.

The Role of Therapy and Counseling

Therapy and counseling can play a vital role in managing hypertension, especially when it's linked to emotional and psychological factors. Professional therapists can help individuals understand and manage their stressors and emotional responses more effectively. Types of therapy beneficial for hypertension include:

- Psychological Counseling:
Helps in identifying stressors and developing coping strategies.
- Behavioral Therapy:
Focuses on changing behaviors that contribute to stress and hypertension, like poor diet or lack of exercise.
- Stress Management
Counseling: Specifically aimed at teaching skills to reduce and manage stress.
- Biofeedback:
A technique that teaches control over certain physiological processes that affect blood pressure, such as heart rate and muscle tension.

Through emotional regulation and stress management, individuals with hypertension can not only manage their blood pressure more effectively but also improve their overall quality of life. The subsequent chapters will continue to explore how integrating these techniques with other lifestyle modifications can offer a comprehensive approach to managing hypertension.

Chapter 8: Diet, Lifestyle, and Hypertension
- The role of diet in managing hypertension.
- Importance of physical activity.
- Lifestyle modifications to support somatic practices
The Role of Diet in Managing Hypertension

- The role of diet in managing hypertension.

Diet plays a crucial role in the management and control of hypertension. Certain foods can increase blood pressure, while others can help to lower it. A diet rich in fruits, vegetables, whole grains, and low-fat dairy products, and low in saturated fat and cholesterol can significantly reduce blood pressure. This dietary approach is often referred to as the Dietary Approaches to Stop Hypertension (DASH) diet.

1. Reducing Sodium Intake:
   High sodium intake is a known contributor to increased blood pressure. The American Heart Association recommends no more than 2,300 milligrams a day, moving toward an ideal limit of no more than 1,500 mg per day for most adults.
2. Increasing Potassium:
   Potassium helps balance the amount of sodium in the cells and can ease tension in the blood vessel walls. Foods rich in potassium include bananas, oranges, cantaloupes, and spinach.
3. Limiting Alcohol and Caffeine:
   Both alcohol and caffeine can raise blood pressure. Moderation is key, and it's often recommended to limit alcohol to one drink a day for women and two for men.
4. Healthy Fats:

Incorporating healthy fats, such as those found in fish, nuts, and olive oil, can also have a beneficial effect on heart health and blood pressure.

Importance of Physical Activity

Regular physical activity is another crucial factor in managing hypertension. Exercise strengthens the heart muscle, improves blood circulation, and helps in maintaining a healthy weight, all of which are essential for lowering and controlling blood pressure.

1. Aerobic Exercise:
   Activities like walking, jogging, cycling, or swimming for at least 150 minutes a week can significantly lower blood pressure.
2. Strength Training:
   Incorporating strength training exercises at least two days a week can also help in reducing blood pressure.
3. Flexibility and Balance Exercises:
   Practices like yoga and Tai Chi not only improve flexibility and balance but also contribute to stress reduction, which is beneficial for blood pressure management.

Lifestyle Modifications to Support Somatic Practices

Integrating somatic practices with specific lifestyle modifications can create a synergistic effect in managing hypertension. Lifestyle changes not only support the physical aspects of health but also enhance the effectiveness of somatic practices.

1. Stress Management:

Adopting techniques such as deep breathing, meditation, or spending time in nature can help manage stress, a significant contributor to hypertension.

2. Regular Sleep Patterns:
   Adequate and quality sleep is vital for overall health and can help in managing blood pressure. Establishing a regular sleep schedule and creating a restful environment can significantly improve sleep quality.

3. Avoiding Tobacco and Limiting Alcohol:
   Smoking and excessive alcohol consumption can adversely affect blood pressure. Quitting smoking and moderating alcohol intake can greatly improve heart health.

4. Healthy Social Interactions:
   Engaging in positive social activities and nurturing supportive relationships can contribute to emotional well-being, which is essential in managing hypertension.

5. Mindful Eating:
   Paying attention to eating habits, such as eating slowly and without distraction, can enhance the effectiveness of dietary changes.

In conclusion, managing hypertension involves a holistic approach that includes dietary changes, regular physical activity, and other lifestyle modifications. These changes not only contribute directly to lowering blood pressure but also enhance the effectiveness of somatic therapies, creating a comprehensive approach to managing hypertension. The next chapters will delve into how to effectively incorporate these changes into daily life, offering practical tips and strategies for long-term success.

Chapter 9: Integrating Somatic Therapy into Daily Life

- Developing a daily somatic routine.
- Overcoming challenges and staying motivated.
- Case studies and success stories.

Developing a Daily Somatic Routine

Incorporating somatic therapy into daily life is a key step in managing hypertension. A daily routine ensures consistency and maximizes the benefits of somatic practices. Here are some tips for developing such a routine:

1. Start Small:
   Begin with simple exercises that can be easily incorporated into your daily schedule, such as mindful breathing or basic stretching.
2. Create a Schedule:
   Set aside a specific time each day for somatic practices. This could be in the morning to energize and prepare for the day or in the evening to unwind.
3. Diverse Techniques:
   Incorporate a variety of techniques, such as yoga, Tai Chi, or body scanning, to keep the routine engaging and cover different aspects of somatic therapy.
4. Mindful Activities:
   Engage in activities that naturally incorporate mindfulness, like walking or gardening, to deepen the practice.
5. Use Technology:
   Apps and online resources can provide guidance and structure, especially for beginners.

Overcoming Challenges and Staying Motivated

Maintaining a somatic routine can be challenging, especially with the busy pace of modern life. Here are strategies to stay motivated:

1. Set Realistic Goals:
   Establish achievable goals and gradually build up the intensity and duration of your somatic practices.
2. Track Progress:
   Keeping a journal or log can help you track progress and notice improvements in your health and well-being.
3. Find a Community:
   Joining a group or class can provide support and motivation. Sharing experiences with others can be encouraging.
4. Flexible Approach:
   Be flexible in your routine. If you miss a session, simply resume the practice without self-judgment.
5. Focus on Benefits:
   Remind yourself of the positive impacts on your health and well-being to stay motivated.

Case Studies and Success Stories

Real-life success stories can be highly motivating and provide insights into the practical application of somatic therapy in managing hypertension.

1. Case Study 1:

A 50-year-old individual with chronic hypertension incorporated daily Tai Chi and mindful breathing into their routine. Over several months, they reported not only a significant drop in blood pressure but also improved stress management and overall well-being.

2. Case Study 2:
   A person experiencing stress-induced hypertension adopted a routine of yoga and guided imagery. This not only helped in lowering their blood pressure but also improved their sleep quality and emotional health.
3. Success Story:
   An individual struggling with hypertension and anxiety found relief through body scanning and progressive muscle relaxation. These practices helped them understand the link between their physical sensations and emotional states, leading to better hypertension management.

These cases illustrate the potential of integrating somatic therapy into daily life for managing hypertension. They highlight the importance of consistency, a holistic approach, and the powerful impact of mind-body practices on health.

In summary, integrating somatic therapy into daily life involves establishing a routine, staying motivated, and learning from others' experiences. This holistic approach to managing hypertension can lead to significant improvements in health and well-being. The final chapter will explore the future directions and emerging research in somatic therapy for hypertension, providing a glimpse into the potential developments in this field.

Chapter 10: Future Directions and Research

- Emerging research in somatic therapy for hypertension.
- Integrating somatic practices with medical treatment.
- The future of holistic approaches to hypertension management.

Emerging Research in Somatic Therapy for Hypertension

The field of somatic therapy is continually evolving, with new research shedding light on its effectiveness in managing hypertension. Emerging studies are focusing on how specific somatic practices can directly influence blood pressure and overall cardiovascular health.

1. Mind-Body Interaction:
   Research is increasingly exploring the intricate connection between psychological processes and physical health, particularly looking at how stress and emotions affect blood pressure.
2. Effectiveness of Specific Techniques:
   Studies are examining which somatic practices are most effective for hypertension, such as comparing different types of meditation or relaxation techniques.
3. Long-Term Effects:
   There is a growing interest in understanding the long-term benefits of somatic practices on hypertension and whether they can sustainably reduce blood pressure over time.
4. Mechanisms of Action:
   Research is delving into the physiological mechanisms through which somatic therapy affects blood pressure, such as its impact on the

autonomic nervous system and stress hormone levels.

Integrating Somatic Practices with Medical Treatment

Integrating somatic practices with traditional medical treatments for hypertension presents a holistic approach to healthcare. This integration is gaining traction in the medical community, with more practitioners recognizing the benefits of a comprehensive treatment plan.

1. Collaborative Care Models:
   Healthcare providers are increasingly adopting models that include both medical treatments and somatic practices, offering a more rounded approach to hypertension management.
2. Patient Education:
   Educating patients about the benefits of somatic practices and how they can complement medical treatments is crucial for this integrated approach.
3. Customized Treatment Plans:
   Future healthcare may see more personalized treatment plans that combine medication, diet, exercise, and specific somatic techniques tailored to individual patient needs.

The Future of Holistic Approaches to Hypertension Management

The future of hypertension management is likely to be more holistic, taking into account the entire individual –

their physical health, mental state, emotional well-being, and lifestyle.

1. Technology and Digital Health:
   The use of digital tools and telehealth services in delivering somatic therapy and tracking patient progress is expected to grow, making these practices more accessible.
2. Preventive Approaches:
   There may be a shift towards preventive measures, incorporating somatic practices early on to manage stress and other risk factors for hypertension.
3. Research and Innovation:
   Ongoing research will likely bring new insights and innovations in somatic therapy, potentially leading to the development of new techniques specifically designed for hypertension management.
4. Public Health Initiatives:
   With the increasing recognition of the benefits of somatic practices, public health initiatives may start to include these therapies as part of broader health promotion campaigns.

In conclusion, the future of managing hypertension lies in a more integrated, patient-centered approach. Somatic therapy, with its focus on the mind-body connection, plays a critical role in this paradigm. As research continues to evolve, it will likely provide a deeper understanding and wider acceptance of somatic practices in hypertension management, heralding a new era in holistic healthcare.

54

Chapter 11. Daily routine recommended

Creating a daily routine of exercises using somatic therapy to improve hypertension involves incorporating practices that focus on relaxation, body awareness, and stress reduction. Here's a detailed routine with specific exercises:

Morning Routine

1. Mindful Breathing (5-10 minutes)
- How to Do It: Sit or lie in a comfortable position. Close your eyes and focus on your natural breathing pattern. Notice the rise and fall of your chest and the sensation of air entering and exiting your nostrils.
- Benefits: This exercise helps activate the parasympathetic nervous system, reducing stress and aiding in lowering blood pressure.

2. Gentle Yoga Stretches (15-20 minutes)
- Specific Poses:
  - Cat-Cow Stretch: On all fours, alternate between arching your back (cat) and lifting your head and tailbone (cow). This helps in spinal flexibility and relaxation.
  - Child's Pose: Sit on your heels, fold forward, and stretch your arms in front of you. It's a restorative pose that calms the mind and relieves tension.
- Benefits: Enhances flexibility, improves circulation, and fosters a state of relaxation, all beneficial for managing hypertension.

Midday Routine

3. Progressive Muscle Relaxation (10-15 minutes)

- How to Do It: Find a quiet place to sit or lie down. Tense each muscle group (starting from the feet and moving upwards) for 5 seconds and then relax for 30 seconds. Pay attention to the contrast between tension and relaxation.
- Benefits: Reduces muscle tension and stress, which can indirectly help lower blood pressure.

4. Mindful Walking (15-20 minutes)
- How to Do It: Walk at a relaxed, slow pace. Focus on the sensation of your feet touching the ground, the rhythm of your walk, and your breathing. If your mind wanders, gently bring your focus back to your walking.
- Benefits: Encourages mindfulness and stress reduction, plus the added cardiovascular benefits of walking.

Evening Routine

5. Guided Imagery or Visualization (10-15 minutes)
- How to Do It: In a quiet and comfortable space, close your eyes, and imagine a peaceful setting (like a beach or forest). Engage all your senses to make the experience as vivid as possible. Use guided imagery recordings if needed.
- Benefits: Reduces stress and anxiety, which are often linked with high blood pressure.

6. Tai Chi or Qigong (20-30 minutes)
- How to Do It: Practice gentle Tai Chi or Qigong movements, focusing on the flow and breath. These practices can often be learned through classes or instructional videos.

- Benefits: These gentle martial arts improve balance, flexibility, and strength, along with reducing stress levels.

Before Bed

7. Body Scanning (5-10 minutes)
- How to Do It: Lie down in bed, close your eyes, and mentally scan your body from head to toe. Notice any areas of tension and consciously relax them.
- Benefits: Promotes relaxation and body awareness, helping in better sleep which is vital for blood pressure regulation.

General Tips:
- Consistency is key. Try to do these exercises daily.
- Listen to your body. If any exercise causes discomfort, modify or skip it.
- Pair this routine with a healthy diet, adequate hydration, and regular medical check-ups.

This routine incorporates a variety of somatic practices targeting different aspects of hypertension, such as stress reduction, increased body awareness, and overall relaxation. It's important to remember that these exercises should complement, not replace, any medical treatment for hypertension. Always consult with a healthcare provider before starting any new exercise regimen, especially if you have health concerns.

Chapter 12. Reference

-Books
-Academic research

Books on Hypertension:

1. "The High Blood Pressure Solution: A Scientifically Proven Program for Preventing Strokes and Heart Disease" by Richard D. Moore, MD, PhD
   - This book offers a comprehensive approach to managing hypertension, providing scientifically backed strategies for preventing strokes and heart disease. It covers lifestyle changes, dietary recommendations, and medication options.

2. "The Complete DASH Diet for Beginners: The Essential Guide to Lowering Blood Pressure and Boosting Your Body's Natural Defenses" by Jennifer Koslo, PhD, RD, CSSD
   - Focused on the DASH (Dietary Approaches to Stop Hypertension) diet, this book provides a beginner-friendly guide to lowering blood pressure through dietary changes. It includes meal plans, recipes, and tips for implementing the DASH diet into daily life.

3. "The High Blood Pressure Hoax" by Sherry A. Rogers, MD
   - Dr. Rogers challenges conventional wisdom about hypertension in this book, offering alternative perspectives on the causes and treatments for high blood pressure. She discusses environmental factors, nutritional approaches, and detoxification strategies.

4. "Thirty Days to Natural Blood Pressure Control: The "No Pressure" Solution" by David DeRose, MD, MPH, and Greg Steinke, MD, MPH
   - This book presents a 30-day program designed to help readers naturally lower their blood pressure. It covers lifestyle modifications, dietary changes, stress management techniques, and exercise routines.

5. "Hypertension Cookbook for Dummies" by Rosanne Rust, MS, RDN, LDN, and Cynthia Kleckner, RDN
   - Geared towards individuals with hypertension, this cookbook offers practical advice and recipes tailored to support blood pressure management. It includes nutritional information, meal plans, and delicious, heart-healthy recipes.

These books cover a range of approaches to understanding and managing hypertension, from dietary interventions to lifestyle modifications and medical considerations. Readers can find guidance on how to effectively control their blood pressure and reduce the risk of associated health complications.)

Books on Somatic Therapy:

Certainly! Here are some books on somatic theory along with brief descriptions of their content:

1. "The Body Keeps the Score: Brain, Mind, and Body in the Healing of Trauma" by Bessel van der Kolk, MD
   - This book explores how trauma affects the body and mind, delving into the role of the nervous system, brain, and physiology in processing and healing traumatic experiences. It offers insights into somatic therapies

and techniques for addressing trauma-related symptoms.

2. "Waking the Tiger: Healing Trauma" by Peter A. Levine, PhD, and Ann Frederick
   - Dr. Peter Levine introduces the concept of somatic experiencing in this book, proposing that trauma is stored in the body and can be released through mindful attention to bodily sensations. He presents case studies and exercises to guide readers through the process of healing trauma.

3. "The Embodied Mind: Cognitive Science and Human Experience" by Francisco J. Varela, Evan Thompson, and Eleanor Rosch
   - This seminal work explores the relationship between mind, body, and consciousness from a cognitive science perspective. It discusses how our embodiment shapes our perception, cognition, and experience, drawing on insights from neuroscience, philosophy, and phenomenology.

4. "In an Unspoken Voice: How the Body Releases Trauma and Restores Goodness" by Peter A. Levine, PhD
   - Building on his previous work, Dr. Peter Levine offers further insights into somatic experiencing and trauma resolution. He explores the role of the body's innate capacity for healing and provides practical exercises for releasing trauma and restoring a sense of wholeness.

5. "Somatic Psychotherapy Toolbox: 125 Worksheets and Exercises to Treat Trauma & Stress" by Manuela Mischke-Reeds, MA, LMFT

- This practical guidebook offers a collection of worksheets and exercises for somatic therapists and clients to use in the treatment of trauma and stress. It covers a wide range of somatic techniques, including mindfulness, body awareness, breathwork, and movement practices.

These books provide valuable insights into somatic theory and its application in understanding and treating trauma, stress, and psychological disorders. They offer a holistic perspective that integrates the body, mind, and emotions, emphasizing the importance of embodied experiences in healing and well-being.

Books on somatic theory and hypertension

1. "The Relaxation Response" by Herbert Benson, MD
 - This classic book introduces the concept of the relaxation response, a physiological state characterized by decreased heart rate, blood pressure, and muscle tension. Dr. Benson explores how practices such as meditation, deep breathing, and progressive muscle relaxation can elicit the relaxation response and promote overall health and well-being, which can indirectly help in managing hypertension.

2. "Full Catastrophe Living: Using the Wisdom of Your Body and Mind to Face Stress, Pain, and Illness" by Jon Kabat-Zinn
 - Jon Kabat-Zinn, founder of the Mindfulness-Based Stress Reduction (MBSR) program, offers insights and practical techniques for using mindfulness to cope with stress, pain, and illness. He emphasizes the importance of paying attention to bodily sensations and cultivating

present-moment awareness as a means of reducing stress and improving overall health.

3. "The Body Keeps the Score: Brain, Mind, and Body in the Healing of Trauma" by Bessel van der Kolk, MD
   - While primarily focused on trauma and its effects on the body and mind, this book by Dr. Bessel van der Kolk explores somatic approaches to healing and well-being. It delves into how trauma can manifest in the body and offers insights into somatic therapies and techniques that can help individuals process and release trauma, which may indirectly contribute to managing conditions like hypertension.

4. "The Healing Power of the Breath: Simple Techniques to Reduce Stress and Anxiety, Enhance Concentration, and Balance Your Emotions" by Richard P. Brown, MD, and Patricia L. Gerbarg, MD
   - Drs. Brown and Gerbarg present a series of breathing techniques derived from yoga and other traditions that promote relaxation, reduce stress, and improve overall health. They discuss the physiological effects of breathing practices on the autonomic nervous system, including its impact on heart rate and blood pressure, offering practical guidance for incorporating breathwork into daily life.

While these books may not directly address hypertension, they offer valuable insights and techniques rooted in somatic principles that can contribute to stress reduction, relaxation, and overall well-being, which are important factors in managing hypertension.

Academic research:

Academic Open Access Journals

Notable open access journals that are known for publishing high-quality, peer-reviewed academic research in various fields. While these journals cover a broad range of topics, many of them include studies related to health, nutrition, medicine, and related sciences, which would encompass research on topics like food and hypertension:

1. PLOS ONE (Public Library of Science ONE)
   - Covers a wide range of scientific disciplines including life sciences, environmental sciences, and health sciences.
(https://www.plosone.org/)

2. BMJ Open
   - An online, open access journal, dedicated to publishing medical research from all disciplines and therapeutic areas.
 (https://bmjopen.bmj.com/)

3. Frontiers
   - A leading open access publisher with journals covering a wide array of academic disciplines, including health, nutrition, and medicine.
 (https://www.frontiersin.org/)

4. BioMed Central (BMC)
   - Offers a large portfolio of peer-reviewed open access journals, encompassing all areas of biology, biomedicine, and medicine.
 (https://www.biomedcentral.com/)

5. MDPI (Multidisciplinary Digital Publishing Institute)
   - Publishes a wide range of open access journals including "Nutrients", which focuses on human nutrition.
(https://www.mdpi.com/)

6. Hindawi
   - Publishes peer-reviewed, open access journals covering a wide range of academic disciplines including medicine and health sciences.
 (https://www.hindawi.com/)

7. eLife
   - An open access journal that publishes research in the life sciences and biomedicine.
 (https://elifesciences.org/)

8. Scientific Reports (Nature Publishing Group)
   - An open access journal publishing original research from all areas of the natural and clinical sciences.
 (https://www.nature.com/srep/)

9. JAMA Network Open
   - An international open access journal publishing clinical care, health policy, and global health research.
(https://jamanetwork.com/journals/jamanetworkopen
)

10. The Lancet Digital Health
   - A gold open access journal in the Lancet family, dedicated to digital health and health informatics.
(https://www.thelancet.com/digital-health)

Searching key words

To search for academic papers or resources in scholarly databases you can use the following keywords and phrases. These will help you narrow down your search to find relevant and scholarly articles, papers, or discussions that relate to the concepts and theories presented in the book:

1. Somatic therapy
2. Body-oriented therapy
3. Body-based therapy
4. Embodied therapy
5. Somatic experiencing
6. Mind-body therapy
7. Body-mind therapy
8. Somatic psychology
9. Somatic awareness
10. Somatic interventions
11. Hypertension
12. High blood pressure
13. Blood pressure regulation
14. Blood pressure management
15. Cardiovascular health and somatic therapy

Using combinations of these keywords in your search queries will help you find relevant academic papers and research studies on the intersection of somatic therapy and hypertension.

Remember to use Boolean operators like "AND" and "OR" to refine your searches further. For instance, "Somatic Theory AND Depression", "Somatic symptoms OR Depression".

THE END